The
Mother
&Child
Project

DISCUSSION GUIDE

The Mother & Child Project

RAISING OUR VOICES *for* HEALTH AND HOPE

DISCUSSION GUIDE

Compiled by
Hope Through Healing Hands

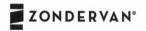

ZONDERVAN

The Mother and Child Project Discussion Guide
Copyright © 2015 by Zondervan

This title is also available as a Zondervan ebook. Visit www.zondervan.com/ebooks.

Requests for information should be addressed to:
Zondervan, 3900 Sparks Dr. SE, Grand Rapids, Michigan 49546

ISBN 978-0-310-34714-9

Cover design: Dual Identity
Cover photography: Esther Havens
Interior design: Kait Lamphere

First Printing February 2015 / Printed in the United States of America

Contents

Introduction

Over the last decade, the church has been at the helm of turning the tide of HIV/AIDS around the world. Today, there is a new focus, a new nexus among global health challenges: maternal, newborn, and child health. *The Mother and Child Project: Raising Our Voices for Health and Hope* is a collection of essays written by artists and actors, nurses and doctors, policymakers and pastors highlighting the spectrum of concerns for mothers and children around the world. This book's goal is to educate readers on the critical importance that healthy timing and spacing of pregnancies (HTSP) plays to:

- combat extreme poverty,
- keep girls and children in school,
- promote gender equality,
- improve maternal and child health,
- and prevent mother-to-child transmission of HIV/AIDS.

We believe that HTSP, or family planning, is at the nexus of global health issues.

This discussion guide will lead you and your group—whether a Sunday school class, community group, small group Bible study, or any other group of individuals—through four weeks of discussion on the issues related to women in the developing world.

Each small group leader has the responsibility to make sure group members know what to read in preparation for their discussion each week. We recommend assigning these readings at least a week before the meeting, to give people ample time to prepare.

Our hope is that these discussions will inspire you to action. We welcome you to research the resources listed in the back of *The Mother and Child Project* for advocacy and involvement, so that you can take part in joining us to help save the lives of millions of mothers and children around the world.

A Call to Compassion

At Home

The concerns surrounding maternal and child health in the developing world are broad and complex, and there are no easy answers to the reasons why millions of women and children die each year from preventable causes. But let's take a look at some facts:

- Every year, more than 287,000 women die in childbirth or from pregnancy-related complications.
- For every woman who dies, there are 30 more who suffer serious illness or debilitating injuries.
- When a mother dies, her child is 10 times more likely to die prematurely. This contributes to the fact that 6.6 million children die each year before their fifth birthday.
- The situation is tragic but not hopeless: 80 percent of maternal deaths are *completely* preventable.

Now that you know the foundation of the problem, let's learn more. Before you meet, read the following essays from part 1 of *The Mother and Child Project*:

- "Miheret Gebrehiwot's Story: Ethiopia"
- "Choosing Joy for Mothers and Children," by Kay Warren
- "All Lives Have Equal Value," by Melinda Gates
- "Contraception Is a Pro-Life Cause in Developing World," by Bill Frist and Jenny Eaton Dyer
- "Family Planning as a Pro-Life Cause," by Michael Gerson
- "A Mama Knows," by Rachel Held Evans

In Your Small Group

Discuss

1. Read Deuteronomy 15:7. How, in your opinion, does this exhortation to care for the poor relate to the discussion of maternal health?

2. Prior to reading these essays, what was your perception of the problems surrounding women's and children's health in the developing world?

   If you have ever seen this problem firsthand, share that experience and what it was like.

3. Look at the photograph of the woman on the front cover of *The Mother and Child Project Discussion Guide*. Think about her life experience and how different it is from your own. In what ways do you imagine it might be similar?

This woman's name is Mpendubundi, and her daughter, now eight years old, was able to attend school for the first time in 2014. Does knowing details about Mpendubundi's life make it harder to ignore her? If so, why do you think this is the case?

4. Review Mihret Gebrehiwot's story. What was the most remarkable aspect of it, in your opinion? How did healthy timing and spacing of pregnancies change the course of Mihret's life?

Last year, more than 6.6 million children under the age of five died from preventable, treatable causes. Many of these children died in the arms of loving parents who simply didn't have access to basic newborn care, simple antibiotics, vaccines, or oral rehydration therapies. For pennies to the dollar, these children's lives could have been saved. In addition, more than 287,000 women died last year in childbirth . . . because they lacked a skilled attendant . . . and had complications during pregnancy or delivery.

Kay Warren

5. What was your response when you first read that more than 6 million newborns and children and 287,000 mothers will die this year? Do you find it hard to grasp how many people that is? (*Note: Imagine yourself at a sold-out football game in a stadium that seats 100,000 people. Then, imagine it filled nearly three times over with mothers who will die, mostly from preventable causes.*)

> We, as Americans, can choose to prevent these deaths with our personal and governmental support for maternal, newborn, and child health and healthy timing and spacing of pregnancies in ways that honor God. Our voices can and will make a difference.
>
> And, in doing so, we choose joy.
>
> *Kay Warren*

6. Do you believe God cares about our reproductive lives? How does providing assistance to mothers for increased maternal, newborn, and child health honor God?

How is it possible to choose joy in the face of such tragic statistics? And how can people of faith be responsible for providing joy to those who are suffering?

7. Why does systemic change take both personal and governmental support? What are the benefits of leveraging governmental funds for these issues? What are the benefits of supporting individually through a nonprofit? What might be the negatives? (*Note: Half of all Americans believe that over 25 percent of the US Budget goes to foreign assistance. Fact: Less than two-thirds of 1 percent (0.6) actually goes to international foreign assistance, and only 25 percent of that to global health.*)

> To help women and children fulfill their potential, we need to make sure they can receive the right kind of health care at every phase of their lives. Each aspect of reproductive, maternal, newborn, and child health connects to the next. To take one example, when women plan for healthy timing and spacing of pregnancies (HTSP), they are more likely to be healthy, and they are more likely to have healthier babies. Healthy babies are more likely to grow up strong and become productive adults. It's a virtuous cycle.
>
> *Melinda Gates*

8. Melinda Gates discusses the "virtuous cycle" of intervening in women's health at each stage of their lives. What do you think she means by "virtuous cycle"?

What can people of faith do to ensure that a virtuous cycle is possible?

> For those of us who identify as pro-life, it's not enough simply to oppose abortion. We must also actively advocate for and invest in actions that save the lives of women and children worldwide.
> *Rachel Held Evans*

9. What does it mean to be "pro-life"? Why is it not enough to simply oppose abortion? What might be a more comprehensive "pro-life" ethic for the world's poorest women and children?

10. Two-hundred and twenty million women in developing nations want to avoid pregnancy but lack the family planning information, education, and resources to do so. What are some consequences of this?

Do you believe Christians should care about women's access to contraception? Why or why not?

When we talk about voluntary family planning in the international context, what do we mean? The definition [we] use is enabling women and couples to determine the number of pregnancies and their timing, and equipping women to use voluntary methods for preventing pregnancy, not including abortion, that are harmonious with their values and beliefs.

Bill Frist and Jenny Eaton Dyer

11. What do you think of when you hear the term "family planning"? (*Note: "Family planning" here includes the broad range of resources—from contraceptives to natural family planning techniques—that help women prevent pregnancy. Family planning does not mean abortion. In fact, the Helms Amendment of 1973 prohibits the use of U.S. governmental foreign assistance funding for abortion. Do you believe this is widely known in the faith community?*)

The words "family planning" light up the limbic centers of American politics. From a distance, it seems like a culture war showdown. Close up, in places such as Bweremana, it is undeniably pro-life.

Michael Gerson

12. What kinds of situations do the women of Bweremana face when delivering their children that we do not typically face in the United States?

13. How does healthy timing and spacing of pregnancies, or "family planning," save lives? And how can we, as people of faith, begin to look "close up" at the importance of global family planning and engage in healthy dialogue on this issue in American politics?

Take Action: Pray

We hope you're inspired and motivated to take action to help the 287,000 women and 6.6 million children who will die this year because they don't have access to the same medical care Westerners do. But before you jump into a plan, take time to think and pray about how God might be calling you to be involved.

Prayer

Lord, give me the knowledge to learn more about the complications of a life lived in extreme poverty. Give me the courage to understand the daily trials of those living in the developing world. And give me the wisdom to know my calling to help the world's most vulnerable — the women and children. Amen.

Healthier Moms, Healthier World

At Home

Before you meet, read the following essays from part 2 of *The Mother and Child Project*:

- "Beryl Anyango's Story: Kenya"
- "Helping Women Isn't Just a 'Nice' Thing to Do," by Hillary Clinton
- "Maternal Health and the Strategy for Empowering Women," by Bruce Wilkinson
- "Better Moms Make a Better World," by Sherry Surratt
- "Healthy Mothers Create Healthy Societies—and a Safer World," by Kay Granger

In Your Small Group

Discuss

1. Read John 10:10. Together as a group, make a list of all the things that are included in having a "full" life.

2. Review the benefits of the healthy timing and spacing of pregnancies (HTSP) mentioned in part 1 of *The Mother and Child Project*. How do these benefits contribute to a better life position for women?

3. Review Beryl Anyango's story. How is a woman's ability to deliver a healthy child tied to her value in the society in which Beryl lives?

> We had to reach out, not only to men, in solidarity and recruit-
> ment, but to religious communities, to every partner we could
> find. We had to make the case to the whole world that creating
> opportunities for women and girls advances security and pros-
> perity for everyone. So we relied on the empirical research that
> shows that when women participate in the economy, everyone
> benefits. When women participate in peace-making and peace-
> keeping, we are all safer and more secure.
>
> *Hillary Clinton*

4. Setting aside your own personal political leanings, discuss this statement from Hillary Clinton from an international perspective. How might developing nations benefit from listening to the experience of women in their desire to grow peace in their regions of the world?

5. Think of places around the world, such as Afghanistan, Pakistan, and Egypt, where women are not allowed to participate as full and equal citizens. How would those countries be better off if women and girls were given more opportunity to contribute to society?

What factors prevent these women and girls from participating in society? How does maternal health and lack of access to contraception play into this?

Mothers are the cornerstones on which families rest. Whether in New York or Nigeria, in the city or the countryside, in a developing or an industrialized nation, a healthy mother can expect to have healthier children.

Bruce Wilkinson

6. Share some examples of how a healthy mother (in every sense of the word) can expect to have healthier children.

Part of this CMMB (Catholic Medical Mission Board) strategy must be dedicated to the empowerment of women. This means economic empowerment, of course, but it also means helping women develop and master the knowledge and tools to manage their own health. Because of the incredible danger associated with too-frequent pregnancy, birth spacing is — and indeed, must be — at the forefront of our approach.

Bruce Wilkinson

7. Discuss the story Bruce Wilkinson shares about the woman in labor who had been educated about birth spacing, which he thinks helped save her own and her child's life. Why is birth spacing at the "forefront" of his organization's approach?

How might birth spacing lead to economic empowerment?

8. Is your church community well positioned to respond to the developing world's maternal health needs? If not, how might you help make that happen?

> As the CEO of MOPS International, I know that moms are a catalyst of health and well-being in the family. After studying the forty years of MOPS Research, I now know what Lillian [a native Kenyan] seemed to instinctively know: moms become better moms when they receive basic training, help, and encouragement, and the impact stretches beyond the walls of the family hut.
>
> *Sherry Surratt*

9. Sherry Surratt notes that "better moms make a better world, one child at a time." How does a woman like Lillian make an impact "beyond the walls of her family hut," effecting change, if she has the knowledge and resources for better health? What does this mean for her involvement in and impact on her community?

10. Compare Monika, from Surratt's essay, "Better Moms Make a Better World," with the woman from Proverbs 31. How are they similar? What challenges does Monica face that we don't see in Proverbs 31?

11. Proverbs 31 says that the good wife's "arms are strong for her tasks" (v. 17 NIV) and "strength and dignity are her clothing, and she smiles at the future" (v. 25 NASB). What are some practical things Christians can do to make a stronger, healthier existence a reality for most women?

Take Action: Share with Friends and Family

This week, continue this discussion with some people from your small group—over the phone, online, or in person. Share what you are reading and discussing on your social networks. If you have a blog, write a post about your thoughts. Commit to talking about this issue at least once during the week, so that your thoughts stay fresh and your inspiration stays ignited. Jot down ideas of ways to help women and children in the developing world, using any insights from *The Mother and Child Project* book as a springboard.

A Day in the Life of a Woman in the Developing World

At Home

Before you meet, read the following essays from part 3 of *The Mother and Child Project*:

- "Namatta Lillian's Story"
- "Kiran Aswathi's Story"
- "What's So Scary About Smart Girls?" by Nicholas Kristof
- "Men as Difference Makers," by James Nardella
- "Too Young to Wed," by Cynthia Gorney
- "Brothels, Survival, and Hope," by Natalie Grant

In Your Small Group

Discuss

1. Read Deuteronomy 10:17 – 18, 27:19; Psalm 146:9; and Proverbs 15:25. What does God promise to do for women?

2. Based on what you've read and learned so far, discuss what the Christian community can do to support women who want access to contraception but don't have it, in order to improve their health and the health of their children?

3. How do you imagine your own life would be different if you had no access to birth control?

   Men, how would your lives be different if your wives had no access to birth control, or if 1 in 39 women in the United States died in childbirth as they do in sub-Saharan Africa? (*Note: In 2013, 28 of every 100,000 women died in childbirth in the United States.*)*

---

* http://data.worldbank.org/indicator/SH.STA.MMRT

4. Review the stories of Namatta and Kiran. How are their lives different? Can you imagine having nine children like Namatta? How might Kiran's life be different if she didn't have access to family planning methods?

Why are fanatics so terrified of girls' education? Because there's no force more powerful to transform a society. The greatest threat to extremism isn't drones firing missiles, but girls reading books . . .

What saddens me is that we in the West aren't acting as rationally. To fight militancy, we invest overwhelmingly in the military toolbox but not so much in the education toolbox that has a far better record at defeating militancy.

Nicholas Kristof

5. Read Daniel 1:17 and Proverbs 1:5. What do those verses tell us about how God feels about children being educated?

What can we as a church or community to do increase girls' access to education in the most backward parts of the world?

6. Ecclesiastes 7:12 says, "Wisdom preserves those who have it" (NIV). How can learning and education preserve the lives of girls (and boys) around the world? What benefits does a child's education have on his or her society?

> The church has the power to influence men as family decision makers and as difference makers between life and death for the women and children in their village communities.
>
> *James Nardella*

7. What difference does it make when men become advocates for healthy timing and spacing of pregnancies? What are steps the church can take, here in America and abroad, to rethink the role of men in family planning and how they contribute to that dialogue to better support the health of their wives and children?

> Child marriage spans continents, language, religion, caste. In India the girls will typically be attached to boys four or five years older; in Yemen, Afghanistan, and other countries with high early-marriage rates, the husbands may be young men or middle-aged widowers or abductors who rape first and claim their victims as wives afterward, as is the practice in certain regions of Ethiopia. Some of these marriages are business transactions, barely adorned with additional rationale: a debt cleared in exchange for an eight-year-old bride; a family feud resolved by the delivery of a virginal twelve-year-old cousin.
>
> *Cynthia Gorney*

8. Cynthia Gorney's exposé on child marriage is tragic but true in many parts of the world. What are some reasons why families may give their young children in marriage? What impact does it have on a girl's life to marry when she's a child?

> The outsider's impulse toward child bride rescue scenarios can be overwhelming: Snatch up the girl, punch out the nearby adults, and run. Just make it stop.
>
> *Cynthia Gorney*

9. How does reading about child marriages cause you to react?

10. Often when we hear of problems so deeply ingrained in certain cultures, we feel nothing *real* can be done to fix them ... and so we do nothing. How can we rise above that attitude and work to bring hope and life to people who are suffering?

I was told by anti-trafficking workers in the field that in many impoverished villages there are almost no children over the age of ten. They are either sent to work in fields, factories, or brothels believing that the "opportunity" will help secure a better future for their families. I personally saw ropes tied to the bedposts in brothels, where women tethered their small children so that they would not crawl away while they worked servicing clients.

Natalie Grant

11. What drives a parent to give up a child to a life of such hopelessness? Do you believe parents are tricked, or has their endemic poverty created a sense of desperation so terrible that it leads them to make heartbreaking decisions for one child in order to protect other children or themselves?

12. In what other ways does poverty destroy families? Discuss the orphans in Moldova and the children tethered to bedposts mentioned in Natalie Grant's essay.

13. When Christ initiated his ministry, he declared that he had come to declare "good news" to the poor (see Matthew 11:5; Luke 4:18). In what way would learning about contraception be good news for a woman living in extreme poverty?

Take Action: Philanthropy

Throughout the next week, start to refine your list of ideas of how you might become involved in this issue. Continue to talk with your group members about what inspires you. Each of the organizations represented in *The Mother and Child Project* were started by a person with a vision, just like you. Join them in their mission, or consider creating a new movement that will reflect God's love to those most vulnerable—the women and children.

Research the organizations working in these fields to see how you can best partner with them through personal service or a financial donation.

How People of Faith Can Help

At Home

Before you meet with your group this week, read the following essays from part 4 of *The Mother and Child Project*:

- "Dorine's Story: Burundi"
- "The Good Samaritan in the Global Village," by Jim Wallis
- "The First-Responder Church," by Santiago "Jimmy" Mellado
- "What Kind of People Ought You to Be?" by Jennie Allen
- "The Old New Thing," by David Dark and Sarah Masen
- "The Village Nearby," by Debbie Dortzbach

In Your Small Group

Discuss

1. Read Micah 6:8, Galatians 6:2, and 3 John 2. What do these verses say is the appropriate Christian response to helping people living in extreme poverty in the developing world?

2. Read Hebrews 6:10 and Psalm 41:1–2. What promise do we have that our work to help mothers and children will not be in vain?

3. Review Dorine's story. How did the church in her community play a role in hindering her health, and how did they help it to thrive?

Helping a man in need by the side of a dangerous road was the example Jesus used to show who our neighbor is and how to help him or her. Who is our neighbor? In our increasingly connected global world, this ancient moral question takes on a whole new context. What does it mean for the Good Samaritan to go global?

Jim Wallis

4. What does it mean for the Good Samaritan to "go global"?

How do modern technologies help us accomplish God's desire to bring justice and mercy to the poor? How can technology help us assist mothers and infants around the world?

It's much easier when our neighbor is a relative, or friend, or member of our group and very much like *us*. But when we have to cross boundaries — like race, religion, neighborhood, region, culture, class, tribe, country, and often gender, even within those other boundaries — the justifications begin for our having ignored somebody or some group of people.

Jim Wallis

5. What justifications have you used to *not* help a neighbor in need?

What are first steps for you or your community "to cross boundaries" to offer help to someone in need? In the case of women in developing nations, what are first steps you can take to aid the "virtuous cycle" and thus save lives and impact communities around the world?

6. Jim Wallis talks about our commitment to the "common good." What does this mean to you? In our highly individualistic society, is it difficult to imagine a generation that would embrace the common good over self-interest? How does the "common good" perspective offer an antidote to narcissism?

> This is where the church can be her best, not because she can do something *for* the poor, but because she will walk closely *with* the poor. There is a world of difference between the two.
> *Santiago "Jimmy" Mellado*

7. What does Jimmy Mellado mean by walking closely "with" the poor?

   How can we grow in "solidarity" with the vulnerable? What position of the heart and mind would that require?

8. In what ways is our relief work unimaginative? How can we be more creative in sharing Jesus's love with the "least of these" in our midst?

Oppression is born of an assumption that women — and usually their children, too — are in some way inferior or have less value than the men around them.

This doesn't begin as formal government action. No governor or dictator says, out of nowhere, that the women in his village or country can't vote or be educated. This oppression begins in our souls. Fears shape our thoughts. Thoughts become culture, and culture defines laws. So when we look out into the world and see oppression of women, we have to remember that it began in the souls of humans. With a belief. With a fear.

Jennie Allen

9. How have you seen fear shape your beliefs and opinions? Has fear caused you to adopt beliefs that might oppress others, even in small ways?

10. What can we do to ensure that we act out of faith in God's plan and provision for all his people, rather than out of fear that our rights will be lost if we work toward a common good? Why is it important to speak up for women's rights?

[We need to be] present enough to the stories of those who suffer for lack of love (and by "love" we mean all that makes for human thriving: enough food and clean water, shelter, good health care, education, safe and beautiful neighborhoods) to recognize Wisdom when she comes knocking on our door. We look up a lot. We ask ourselves, "What are we missing? Who are we marginalizing when we say what we say? Are we using language of exclusion or embrace?"

David Dark and Sarah Masen

11. Is it hard for you to hear stories of suffering, especially when they apply to women and children? Why do you think it's so difficult? How does this shape your perspective about how God relates to suffering?

Think about the language you use when you talk about people who live in extreme poverty. What words do you use? Do they shape your heart more toward exclusion or embrace?

The account in the Gospels* of the bleeding woman healed by Jesus demonstrates the intrinsic worth God sees in women. The unnamed woman, bleeding for twelve years, was stigmatized, spiritually ostracized, extremely weak, and economically impoverished. Yet, drawn by the working of Christ in her life, she ventured into crowded social space and touched Jesus. He cared so deeply and so thoroughly for her that he allowed her blood-impure status to spiritually defile him. It instantly healed the woman.

Debbie Dortzbach

12. Jesus cared enough about the hemorrhaging woman's health and well-being to risk becoming defiled—according to Jewish law—by her. Spend a few moments comparing that act to what he did for us on the cross. (*Can there be any doubt he loves, treasures, honors, and redeems women and seeks to bring his redemption and completeness to all humankind in brokenness and suffering?*)

---

*Matthew 9:20–22; Mark 5:25–34; Luke 8:43–48.

13. If Jesus were on earth today, what do you think he would say about the way the church has responded to women in crisis around the globe? Is our legacy that we truly loved well?

Today, what is your response to God at work in the world and in your life? What "village" is near you, and what are you doing within it?

Take Action: Advocacy

The goal of this book and study has been to broaden our perspective, to learn more about the lives of women and children around the world, and to take part in being the change we want to see in the world.

Now that you've spent four weeks talking about these issues and researching the aspects that are most meaningful to you, what is your plan moving forward? How will you become involved? Set some goals for yourself and be sure to build a support team to help you accomplish them.

One critical way to help is through advocacy (see the Resources section in *The Mother and Child Project*). We ask that you consider lending your voice to "speak up for those who cannot speak for themselves" (Proverbs 31:8 NIV). Consider writing your congressional leaders, letting them know that you care deeply about the lives of women and children in poor countries and that you want to increase funding for maternal, newborn, and child health and healthy timing and spacing of pregnancies. Your voice will make a difference. And united, we may unleash additional governmental funding that will save the lives of millions.

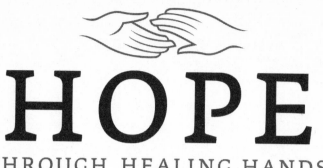

HOPE

THROUGH HEALING HANDS

Hope Through Healing Hands is a nonprofit 501(c)3 whose mission is to promote an improved quality of life for citizens and communities around the world using health as a currency for peace.

Through the prism of health diplomacy, we envision a world where all individuals and families can obtain access to health care information, services, and support for the opportunity at a fuller life. Specifically, we seek sustainability through health care service and training.

This includes efforts for maternal, newborn, and child health; healthy timing and spacing of pregnancies; clean water; extreme poverty; emergency relief; and global diseases such as HIV/AIDS, tuberculosis, and malaria. Strategically, we encourage global health partnerships by working hand in hand with leading organizations that best address these issues in developing nations.

Follow us at:

www.HopeThroughHealingHands.org

@HTHHglobal on Twitter

www.facebook.com/HopeThroughHealingHands

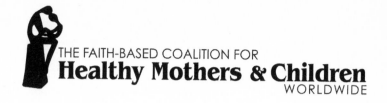

THE FAITH-BASED COALITION FOR
Healthy Mothers & Children
WORLDWIDE

The Faith-Based Coalition for Healthy Mothers and Children Worldwide is a campaign of Hope Through Healing Hands to build a coalition of advocates who are speaking out about the struggles that mothers and children in developing nations face daily. For instance, over 287,000 women in developing nations die from preventable complications during pregnancy and childbirth, and 6.6 million children die from preventable causes before their fifth birthday each year. But we can change this. We seek to galvanize faith-based leaders and their constituencies around the issues of maternal, newborn, and child health (MNCH) as well as healthy timing and spacing of pregnancies (HTSP) to improve maternal health and reduce child mortality.

Our goal is to educate and activate thought-leaders to discuss, debate, and advocate on these issues, addressing MNCH and HTSP. Members of the coalition have varied positions on particular methods, which include fertility-awareness approaches as well as contraceptives, but all agree that healthy timing and spacing of pregnancies is imperative for saving the lives of women and children and enhancing the flourishing of families worldwide.

Join us to learn more about how you can become involved as an advocate for mothers and children. www.hopethroughhealinghands.org/faith-based-coalition